Silent as the Falling Snow

My experience with bowel cancer

John Webb

My thanks to Kaye Rogers for her attention to detail and her patience in editing this story.

I would also like to thank my wife Katherine; who has supported me throughout this journey, encouraged me to write this personal account and provided valuable input.

Self-Published in paperback in Great Britain 2019

Preface

This is a short personal story about my experiences with bowel cancer. It is an account from the time of realising something was wrong, to referrals, undergoing investigations, diagnosis and treatment. I have included the physical and emotional aspects of my condition as well as the processes that begin once we have a medical problem such as bowel cancer. This short story is framed around an 18-month period. I have mentioned everything that was going on at this time, because we do not exist in isolation. No matter what events take place for us as individuals, life goes on around us; the good, the bad and the ugly, including for me, the worry of my son's fight with kidney failure compared to the joy of my wife being presented with the Dr Kate Granger award for compassionate care. This small book is aimed to be informative, sometimes humorous I hope, but above all to give insight into the thoughts, feelings and journey of a cancer sufferer. It aims to demystify the procedures, surgery and chemotherapy involved, hopefully accurately, but is written by someone who is not medically qualified. My aim is to give hope to those diagnosed with bowel cancer or those who wonder what it is like to have a cancer diagnosis. I will forever be indebted to the fast and competent actions of my wife and the amazing skills of my colorectal surgeon, Professor Mark Coleman. I would also like to thank the gastroenterologist, who identified the tumour, those who carried out the scans and interpreted them, the nurses who looked after me, the oncology team who monitored and administered my chemo and all friends and relatives for their emotional support.

I cannot fault my care in the NHS; in my opinion it remains a wonderful institution, my care has been exemplary, and I owe a huge debt to all of the above.

To Katherine Webb, whose insight and prompt actions probably saved my life.

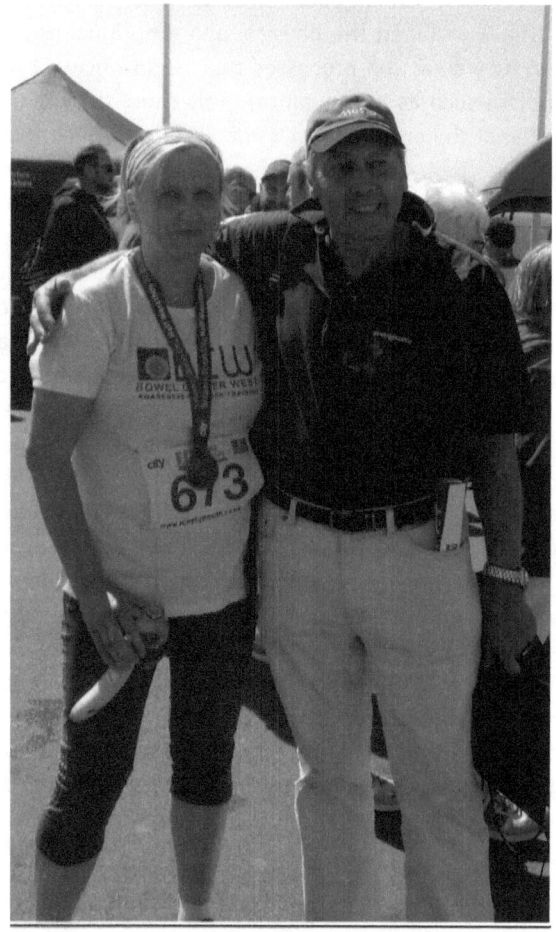

The Plymouth Half Marathon

Silent as the Falling Snow

The grey skies have foreboding told
As winter snow starts to unfold.
Snow's silent creeping flakes appear
And cover all both far and near.

Snow changes all to monochrome
As the sky silently spews its foam.
Depth increasing without sound,
The silent white is all around.

How it makes the landscape change,
Never permanent, just rearranged.
Snow gathers at a fastening speed
And all succumb to its insatiable greed.

John Webb

The Cotswolds

I begin this personal story in early December 2017. My wife, Kathy, and I, together with our beloved Irish Setter, Cara, had travelled from our home on the edge of Dartmoor to Bourton-on-the-Hill in the Cotswolds. I had spent three years in the early 1980s living in the Cotswolds, in a small village near Swinbrook. I still held this lovely part of England in great affection and Kathy and I would revisit this unique part of the country on an annual basis. I have particularly fond memories of taking Lyndon and Samantha my children, who were seven and eight years old, on fishing trips to the river Windrush, which ran through our village. We were restricted to a small area of the riverbank owned by the local farmer as the Cotswold Flyfishers, had exclusive rights along most of the river, if we ever encountered any of the members, they would always make that very point. We never caught any trout large enough to be removed and were quite content to release the young fish we did catch back into the river hoping they would live to a ripe old age. We would also wade into the shallower areas lifting stones and finding the indigenous White Clawed Crayfish, some growing up to five inches in length, their presence an indication of the clean state of the river. They are a delicacy, and I understand are now much in decline due to a fungal disease spread by a non-native North American Signal crayfish,not due to our activities I can assure you. It was a great area to bring up young children, lots of natural habitat to explore and it always felt very safe. Our village Asthall, with a population of about fifty, was made famous by the Mitford sisters, who had spent some seven years living in the Manor House, when their father Baron Redesdale had moved there during the 1st world war. Our small 18c abode built of Cotswold slate was known as Walnut Cottage, we bought it for the princely sum of £30k in 1982 and noted it had sold in 2008 for £750K. Ever felt you had missed an opportunity? At one time it housed Baron Redesdale's groom and chauffeur during the Mitford's tenure. Just opposite Walnut Cottage was a very nice Inn called the Maytime, which my then wife and I frequented. A regular at the Inn was Joe Walker, a retired farmer and relative of the Walker family who owned a two hundred plus acre dairy farm. Joe had his own bar stool in the pub and had lived his entire life in the village. He had played with the young Mitfords in those far off days and was visited during our period living there, by Deborah, who was the Duchess of Devonshire. She was writing a biography and wanted to catch up with him; hopefully for sentimental reasons as well as confirming some detail for her book. Joe had never visited London in his lifetime and had only ever travelled as far as Oxford some seventeen miles away! Who could blame him, it is a special place and whenever Kathy and I visit the Maytime Inn at Asthall I still think of him sitting on that barstool, with his wonderful broad Oxfordshire accent, citing countryside wisdom.

Getting back to our trip to Bourton on the Hill; early December seemed a good time to take a short break before all the Christmas festivities. The two-bedroomed sixteenth-century Cotswold stone cottage we had booked for four nights looked right up our street, with an inglenook fireplace and wood burner. We pictured a few cosy nights in and the not infrequent trip to the local gastropub, a short walk away.

To make the occasion even more atmospheric, it had started snowing as we neared the end of our journey. Leaving the M5 near Gloucester, the area was transformed into something quite magical. As we approached the village, we were not disappointed in the location. The cottage was on a minor road in a very quiet location and Kathy, being a lover of the white stuff, was over the moon as several inches of snow began to settle. Snow falling silently, no sound announcing its arrival or warnings of how deep it may grow.

Once settled into our temporary home, we found a nice walk for Cara across some nearby fields. Having been cooped up in the car for several hours, she made the most of her new-found freedom and was over the moon at this strange white material, snow being a comparatively rare occurrence where we live. She found it was great for digging holes in, snuffling your nose into, and generally sliding around and having fun.

That evening we decided we would sample the gastronomic delights at our local, the Horse and Groom, not to mention an ale or two for me and a couple of glasses of wine for Kathy.

I decided to have fish and chips; not very imaginative but I just fancied it, and Kathy had a chicken dish, both of which were very tasty and well-prepared. The pub was fairly quiet, which probably had a lot to do with the weather and after a couple of hours we returned to our cottage feeling comfortably full and ready for a good night's sleep. Slipping and sliding our way home, the effects no doubt of a combination of snow and alcohol, somehow added to the whole experience. Once home, we wasted no time in retiring to bed and were soon fast asleep.

The following day was Sunday and we were awoken by someone knocking at our front door. It was early for us, about 7.30am, and we had hoped for a bit of a lie-in, as Sunday convention normally dictates. However, on opening the door a lady asked if we might be responsible for blocking her car in. More heavy snow had fallen overnight and although she had a four-wheel drive vehicle, the combination of someone parking very close to her car and snow made her potential exit a hazardous task in a narrow lane. We pleaded not guilty and suggested she try some of the other neighbouring cottages. I asked if there was an urgency for her to drive so early, as probably in an hour or so there might be more people around to lend a hand. She said her horse needed feeding.

I thought, "Never mind waking us up and heaven forbid another hour or so could prove fatal for the four-legged creature, who might starve to death!"

That day we drove to Broadway, as Kathy hadn't been there before, and it is on my list of must-see Cotswold villages. The main roads had been salted and bulldozers were keeping the roads open for traffic. We walked around the shops, had a coffee, then had a snack and picked up some provisions to keep us going for the next few days. Kathy decided she would prepare a cottage pie in the evening, which seemed ideal on a cold winter's night. Before leaving the town, I suggested we have a glass of something in the five-star Lygon Arms. We had a small glass of prosecco each and when the waiter said, "That will be £16", I must have looked a bit shaken. Don't get me wrong, it is a lovely hotel and I had fond memories of staying there in the 1980s, but it didn't pass my notice that we could have bought two decent bottles of wine for that amount. We left after half an hour and arrived back at our

9

now snow-encrusted temporary home. Kathy set about preparing the pie-of-all-pies and I proceeded to lay up the log fire. We decided to have a pre-dinner drink at the Horse and Groom, taking Cara with us as she doesn't like to be left out! The pub looked delightful with its tree and tasteful decorations. There were more customers this evening than the previous night, as the main roads had been cleared and the atmosphere inside was very jovial. Cara received lots of attention from the customers, which she loved. Later, as some very tasty looking meals started arriving on tables, we realised how hungry we were and that it was time for us to head back. Cara would have to forgo further attention by the dog-friendly customers.

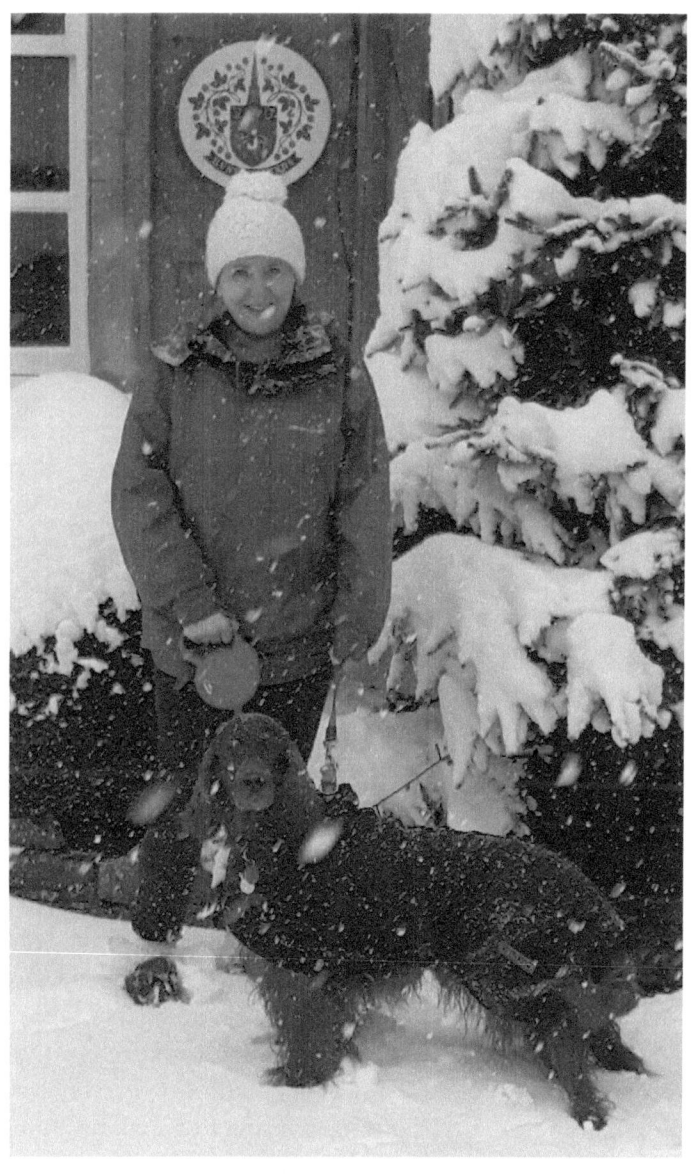

Kathy and Cara outside the Horse and Groom

Once home, I lit the fire and Kathy served up the pie, which looked amazing. I am sure I even had a second helping. We played a few rounds of cards after dinner and had a night cap in front of the glowing fire. We thought it had been a good start to our winter break and the snow an unexpected bonus. Little did we realise we were going to be in for a very disturbed night.

We got off to sleep quite well, but at about midnight I awoke with dreadful abdominal pain. I rarely suffer with any tummy problems; Kathy often says I have a cast iron gut, and she should know as she is the lead nurse for Inflammatory Bowel Disease at our local hospital. The discomfort and noise associated with this episode was quite unlike anything I had experienced before. In the early hours, I had to charge into the bathroom and had a bout of profuse diarrhoea; I will leave that to your imagination. Surely it couldn't be Kathy's cottage pie? She is an excellent cook and anyway it would be too soon after eating. The discomfort and noise in my stomach continued throughout the night. Oddly I had experienced diarrhoea accompanied with vomiting about six weeks before, following a meal out. It was a one-off episode and we had both put this down to food poisoning, but strange that it should happen again.

Eventually by morning I was feeling exhausted, but at least things had calmed down and trips to the bathroom had ceased, but I did look very bloated and had trouble getting my trousers done up! Kathy now looked quite concerned about the whole event. I just thought that it was another case of upset stomach due to something I had eaten during the past 24 hours - maybe that lunchtime snack in Broadway, and it probably had nothing to do with the pie. What I did not know at the time was that when Kathy took Cara for her early morning walk, she had phoned her mother upset and convinced it was something serious. She even said to her mother she thought I might have a tumour that was obstructing the bowel! Her mother, a retired matron, had reassured her that this was surely unlikely and there was probably a much simpler and far less sinister explanation. I knew Kathy had been concerned but didn't know she had been so upset over the events. I also never heard about that conversation she had had with her mother until a couple of weeks later. I had only light meals for the last couple of days of our stay, as I did not want a repeat performance in the bathroom. We had a trip to Burford on one of the days, where I have many fond memories. Lyndon and Samantha had attended the local primary school when we were living in Asthall. I had also taken the boys at the school for football training in a period between my finishing a job with a Swedish manufacturer of disposable operating theatre products and starting another with a subsidiary of an American pharmaceutical company. I suppose being quite nostalgic, when visiting Burford, I would think about those far off days, now some thirty-five years ago. I had really enjoyed my time working for the Swedish company, spending most of it in operating theatres in the many NHS London teaching hospitals and private sector. I still regard it as a privilege, the time I spent watching some of the country's leading surgeons in Orthopaedics and Cancer doing what they did best. However, my overriding memory related to a management team building meeting that our MD had organised in France in 1982. I say, "Team Building", it was effectively to crew on his Maxi Swedish sailing boat, taking it from La Rochelle to

Capbreton across the Bay of Biscay. There were four of us including our Norwegian MD, who was the only experienced sailor amongst us. In fact, none of his crew had ever embarked on a long sailing trip before! The event started with a flight out to Bordeaux and then a 2hr drive to La Rochelle. This was my first trip to this wonderful old city in south western France and I felt excited about our few days in this area and about the time we would spend together on board the yacht. After lunch washed down with the obligatory couple of bottles of Saint-Emilion, we went down to the marina and loaded our gear on board the boat. We familiarised ourselves with our berths that were to be our sleeping quarters and what was to be our home for the next 24 hours or so. My berth was a double in the stern of the boat, which was private and looked comfortable. We then paid a trip to the local Super Marché, where we filled a trolley. I noted that the ratio of alcohol to food in the trolley was probably about 4:1: obviously a portent of things to come. Having returned to the boat and stowed our provisions, we were given a safety briefing and then set about preparing our dinner. The weather was fantastic, clear blue skies and lots of very warm sunshine and having eaten our meal we prepared to leave La Rochelle at about 19.00hrs.

As we sailed away from what is quite a stunning setting, we toasted our safe passage and continued toasting into the small hours, with much hilarity and joking about the reputation of Biscay. After sunset, I had noticed lightning strikes in the far distance, despite drawing this to the attention of my crew members, they laughed and suggested that I might be hallucinating as a result of consuming too many beers. I eventually decided to retire to my berth and left the others still drinking, grateful for the relative privacy and quiet of my sleeping quarters. I should point out that our MD and skipper had helmed the boat since leaving port, throughout the hours of darkness and into the next morning. On waking I joined him in the cockpit and made coffee for him and fellow crew as they emerged one by one from their cocoons. The weather was still stunning and the wind favourable, allowing us to make a good 8 knots of boat speed on a beam reach. We were making good progress towards Capbreton when out of the blue a French naval vessel appeared and contacted us on the VHF advising us to change course, as there was an imminent exercise involving high speed jets in our area. Our skipper made the alteration to our course, which would now add a couple of hours to our journey time. Suddenly a mirage jet appeared and fired a missile at a target a few miles distant. It was a sobering experience and although relieved that we had been warned by the French navy, a quietness descended amongst us. When we set out, we had not expected to be used for target practice by the French air force! We soon forgot the close encounter and enjoyed some cheese and French loaf that we had bought the previous day for our lunch. We continued to revel in the excellent sailing as our yacht cut through the water at a good pace. When very unexpectedly, things changed rapidly. The wind started to back* and the sails needed trimming. The wind now felt very hot almost as though someone had pointed a giant hairdryer at us, it was now coming off the land.

---

* when a depression approaches the wind direction changes in an anti-clockwise direction.

I now know it's called a Scirocco and its origins are in North Africa. The wind strength started to build and within half an hour we were in a full gale with 40 knots. The Bay of Biscay really was living up to its reputation. All our bravado the previous night, fuelled no doubt by wine and beer was now put into a different context. Our genoa (front sail) had torn as we attempted to get it down. Once we had reduced the mainsail, we put the engine on to improve our ability to maintain some speed. Waves were crashing over the boat as we were raised and lowered from peaks to troughs by some twenty feet and we had gone from shorts and T shirts to waterproofs. We all felt sea-sick and we all were very sick, over the boat and often over each other unintentionally. Our skipper was now exhausted having been at the wheel for 20 hours or so. He set a course and one of our crew took the helm. The skipper went below to sleep in the saloon, which I could understand but leaving us in control was not without risk. The combination of reduced sail and motor would have to endure until we reached our destination. An hour or so later we approached the entrance to Capbreton, we woke our skipper; how he had managed to sleep with all the crashing of the boat off the waves into deep troughs I will never know. He would have to pilot us into the harbour; however, he was unsure as to how safe it would be to enter in such rough conditions. The entrance was very narrow, rocks strategically and menacingly arranged on either side, waves breaking at the harbour entrance. A crowd of French people had gathered on the walls by the entrance looking in disbelief at our proposed entry. At the last minute our skipper decided it was too risky and aborted our entry. We would have to sail further south for another 2 hours in the gale to Bayonne, further down the coast for a safer port of entry. He set a new course and he returned to his berth, leaving us novices to take it in terms to helm whilst simultaneously throwing up our lunch, beers and everything else we had consumed in the last 24 hrs. We did eventually arrive at Bayonne, which had a much less risky entrance; our skipper was awake to steer us onto our mooring and we all sighed a sense of relief mixed with exhaustion. As we tied the boat up, our MD said that he was not impressed with the state of his boat cockpit and its revolting contents and I noted he had not succumbed to sickness at any point, but he did congratulate us for our endeavours. We later learned of the lifeboat having to rescue another yacht and of other boats sustaining broken masts from the adverse conditions. It had not escaped my notice that altering our course to avoid the naval exercise had put us at risk in a gale that we otherwise might have avoided. However, the prospect of being blown up by a missile would have been a price too high to pay. With hindsight the liberal use of alcohol, was at best a risky strategy during a challenging journey and I would advise moderation to any embarking on similar adventures.

This was my first real sailing adventure and certainly one of the scariest I have experienced; despite everything it whetted my appetite to sailing, which would become a big part of my future life over the next thirty-five years.

However, as our holiday break neared its end, I was pleased that I had no further bowel discomfort or symptoms. On the morning of our departure, we had to help other residents shovel the road clear of snow in order to get our car out, as a further fall of snow during the night had made driving matters worse.

I must admit I was exhausted after the effort involved, more so than I would normally have expected, but I put it down to my still recovering from those explosive events of our second evening.

Investigations

When we returned to Devon, Kathy said we should drive straight to Derriford hospital in Plymouth. She was so concerned she had arranged for me to have my bloods taken. Within a couple of days, the blood results confirmed I was anaemic and my ferritin, a measure of iron reserves, showed I had been losing blood for some time. This probably explained my tiredness of late and especially after the snow shovelling. When someone of my age, 70 years old at the time, is found to be anaemic it is often recommended you have a colonoscopy. A camera is inserted up your rear end and can then explore the large bowel, known as the colon. The colon is about 5ft long and about 3 inches in diameter. Within 10 days of returning from our trip to the Cotswolds, I had had bloods done and was now about to have both a colonoscopy and a gastroscopy, less than two weeks before Christmas! Things were moving at a pace, primarily as Kathy had many contacts in the gastroenterology department. I must admit I was more concerned about the gastroscopy than the colonoscopy. The idea of having a camera passed down my throat whilst awake seemed much more alarming. In the event, both procedures were conducted by a skilled gastroenterologist and neither was that uncomfortable or scary. Both procedures were conducted with me lying on a table and a TV monitor next to me enabled the consultant to view the progress of the camera either down the oesophagus into the stomach or up the rectum and along the colon. It felt as though I was under attack from both ends, but it was a relief to know that these investigations were under way.

The gastroscopy showed that I had a significant hiatus hernia, where the stomach protrudes above the diaphragm. It is not uncommon; many people cope without too many problems. That, however, was not the cause of my explosive event in the Cotswolds. I had known about the hernia since having a chest x-ray previously, following a bout of pneumonia. It was rarely responsible for any significant problems such as reflux; it did account for gurgling noises, when I was lying down, a cause for other people's amusement.

After the procedures, I got changed and Kathy and I were called into a private waiting room. I didn't think anything was untoward, but Kathy tells me she instantly knew something was wrong because if things are all normal you don't get called into a separate room for a chat, you just get sent on your way! The consultant sat down with us and said that the gastroscopy was fine, other than the hernia. He then explained that the colonoscopy had not been easy (I had a loopy colon, whatever that means) and that at the end of the colon, where it joins the small bowel, called the caecum, he had found a growth. His words were: "It's a tumour and it is cancer." You never want to hear those words; it is always someone else you know or hear about that gets it. I didn't react, however. The consultant continued saying that the tumour was about three inches in size and had probably been growing there for a long time. I remember hearing that a caecal tumour is sometimes called the silent killer, due often to an absence of symptoms, so no warning of its beginnings or subsequent development.

I asked how this could be, as I had only submitted the biannual 'poo test' a few months earlier and it had come back as negative.

The consultant replied that the test is not 100% and does sometimes miss tumours. The poo test I took, acronym gFOB, which stands for guaiac faecal occult blood test, is only taken up by about 60% of the population and misses 30-50% of cancer cases, I know that now!

It is based on someone observing a subjective colour change when testing the stool sample. Although not that sensitive a test, the argument has always been that it has accounted for a 16% reduction in colorectal deaths.

The new poo test, acronym FIT, which stands for faecal immunochemical test, is likely to be more sensitive and because it is easier to conduct, more people are expected to complete the test. The stool sample is tested by a machine analyser, which generates a numerical result for faecal occult blood in micrograms, eliminating much of the human error. However, it is important that anyone with symptoms of a change in bowel habits, including diarrhoea, blood in the stools without other piles (haemorrhoids) symptoms, abdominal pain, discomfort or bloating brought on by eating, should seek medical attention even if they have had a recent negative test result.

Strange to hear the word cancer related to myself, yet oddly I did not feel anything, almost as though it was a relief to know what was wrong. Our bodies are made up of about 35 trillion cells and each cell receives chemical signals which direct and control their actions, including when to divide and multiply, and even when to die. It only takes one wrong signal to one cell to start a cancer. I had seen my mother die from cancer when she was only 63. She had a tumour in her breast and had a radical mastectomy, but two years later the cancer had metastasised and was everywhere; she died soon afterwards. Her death was not pleasant, particularly in the early 70s when palliative care was not as it is now. Witnessing her final days had left a mark on me. So why wasn't I in shock or feeling emotional? I have no single explanation and I am sure in the same situation everyone will react differently. It may be for a combination of reasons that I took the news better than you might expect. Having an interest in Buddhism, getting to know a Tibetan lama and attending many teachings some years ago, I accept that everything is impermanent, including our lives. People often live their lives as though they were going to be around forever. I had also seen at close hand the suffering of others in hospital throughout my career in the pharmaceutical industry and since retiring, in a part-time job with the out-of-hours GP services. I would often drive doctors to see patients in palliative care, some as a result of brain, lung, breast or bowel cancers, to name but a few. I had a good idea of the progression of cancer in such unfortunate patients and the ending they must endure, sometimes as people half my age. I suppose being exposed to all this does influence how I had responded to the news I had been given. However, we are all different and our life experiences may well influence our reaction to a cancer diagnosis. Don't think for one moment that deep down I wasn't also feeling vulnerable and a bit scared; when it's you or someone you know well or love, it is a whole different ball game.

One thing I was to learn over the coming weeks and months was that people react very differently to someone having cancer. I was to find that many people would ask how I was, they would want to know about my disease and its treatment. However, even some people we knew quite well would say nothing about my cancer or ask how I was despite knowing about it. It can seem a bit odd not to be asked how you are feeling, particularly with something potentially life threatening. It's not like we are talking about someone with a cold! Maybe they simply do not know what to say or how to deal with it, or maybe they are just unfeeling individuals. I would hope it's the former.

Having Kathy by my side at this time was my greatest asset; she is a fantastic nurse and a loving wife. I just wonder how I would have coped if she wasn't around. She just seems to know how to deal with all this stuff. I suppose because of her job it becomes second nature. It also made me appreciate the way people without a spouse or partner must cope on their own with a cancer diagnosis. It really must take great strength and I take my hat off to them. I also cannot overstate the advantage of having a wife who knew all the consultants and other healthcare professionals involved. I appreciate most people don't have that, but right now I felt I needed some advantages for what lay ahead.

It was only now that Kathy revealed the conversation she had had with her mother whilst we were away, saying she thought I had an obstructing tumour. She had spoken at length with her mum, crying whilst on her mobile phone, in a field full of snow, Cara racing around enjoying herself unaware of events. I could not believe how she could have made that diagnosis on the basis of what had happened the previous night, but she had got it dead right, even though she admits herself that she told herself she was just being paranoid.

So, I had an advanced tumour and would need radical surgery to remove that big bastard (excuse my French).

I would also need a CT Scan (computerised tomography) prior to an appointment with the colorectal surgeon. The scan takes a series of x-ray pictures, showing cross-sectional slices of your body.

Two days before having the CT scan, you must have a strong laxative (oh great, more bowel evacuation!) This is to totally empty your bowels, so that the scan has an uninterrupted view. It is usually a lemon tasting sachet of sodium picosulphate that you dissolve in water. The effect is quite profound as it causes dramatic emptying of your entire bowel contents. It's not the most pleasant experience, but it's bearable and necessary. Once you have taken the medicine you need to be at home, for obvious reasons.

On meeting Professor Coleman for the first time, he was very charismatic and had a reassuringly confident manner. I had heard about his excellent reputation from Kathy and knew he had trained many years previously with a renowned pioneer in colorectal surgery, Professor "Bill" Heald. I had the pleasure of first meeting Professor Heald in the mid-70s, during the course of my work. The surgeon stated that the operation would be a right-sided hemicolectomy. The tumour had grown through the wall of my colon. The surgery would involve removing about half of my colon, from the caecum where the tumour was located, to mid-way along the transverse colon.

I was thinking feet and inches, that's at least a couple of feet, seems a lot for a tumour that's only three inches but I am sure he has done this countless time and knows what he is doing! He said, on a positive note, that the CT scan had not identified any metastases in the liver or other major organs. That was a relief. I knew if it had spread to other organs, my survival chances would be greatly reduced. He then said he must point out there is always a small risk, with any surgery and a general anaesthetic, of dying on the operating table, I may have a bleed and haemorrhage to death, I could get a blood clot and (not uncommonly) cancer patients post-operatively suffer depression. Well, how reassuring was that! Depression was the last thing on my mind right now, but I could see how later, when given thinking time, it could become an issue. I then realised that it's not just about removing that alien beast from your colon, it's potentially a life-changing diagnosis, affecting you mentally as well as physically, with the ability to shake your being to the core. That's what makes the word CANCER so fearful, life-threatening and life-changing and, in fairness to the surgeon, he had to point out what could happen.

The surgeon said my operation would be in two, weeks' time on the 5th January, all being well, and that it was likely to be followed up with several months of chemotherapy. The medical team would know more after pathology had examined the excised bowel. He said I should stick to a low residue diet in the meantime to avoid any risk of the bowel obstructing and possibly bursting, causing peritonitis. We left the hospital and, although having just heard explicit instructions to follow a low residue diet, I really fancied a burger and chips, which I rarely eat. I just felt in need of a tasty treat after all the news. Kathy reflected humorously how patients often don't adhere to the advice of their clinicians! She did agree to take me for my treat however; it was a small burger and I didn't suffer any ill effects!

I had a rather more subdued Christmas than normal with small meals and generally less snacking. I was very upset that I couldn't have Brussel sprouts, stuffing or Christmas pudding! I did think over this festive period about my diagnosis and what was in store. I also for the first time considered my mortality and even looked at all my finances, making a list for Kathy, just in case. I stuck to the restricted food intake, as I didn't want to risk anything this close to surgery.

I also had concerns that the operation might get cancelled, as at the time the hospital was cancelling a lot of operations due to it being on the highest alert level, now called 'Opel 4'. This is generally when there are no beds available; full occupancy. I would not know until the day, so just kept telling myself that surely, they wouldn't cancel a cancer case.

One important thing going on throughout this whole period, that I have so far not mentioned, involved my son. He was now in his 40s and, in his early 20s, had been diagnosed with polycystic kidneys. This is a chronic condition that ultimately leads to renal failure with all the implications of dialysis and hopefully a kidney transplant or, in the worst case, can lead to an early death. He had lived a normal life thus far, albeit on a regime of multiple antihypertensives to control his high blood pressure as a result of his condition. His attitude had always been positive, knowing that he had a sword hanging over him, that one day would mean operations, dialysis and trying to find a kidney donor in the future. Both his mother and I had also had to wrestle with the worry, knowing life would have to change for him significantly at some stage, whilst still a young man. However, over the past six months, he had been admitted to hospital on several occasions with acute infections in one of his kidneys and had to be treated with intravenous (IV) antibiotics. He was also becoming less well generally, as a result of his kidneys failing and was physically finding life difficult as the kidneys had grown massively due to the formation of numerous cysts. We knew the time was coming when he would have his diseased kidneys removed and would then go onto dialysis. I had driven to Dorchester Hospital just two days prior to my operation to see how he was, knowing it would be a little while before I would be able to make the journey again.

I stayed overnight in a lovely old inn, 'The Greyhound', in a pretty village called Sydling St Nicholas, not far from Dorchester. I did not feel up to a return journey from Plymouth to Dorchester in one day, some four hours' drive. It would be an opportunity to see my son again in the morning, before driving home, and a chance to stay in a lovely inn. You may notice a theme of pubs, inns and real ale. I have to plead guilty to enjoying that particular avenue of pleasure. When settling the bill, the owner of the inn asked if I was doing anything nice. I told him about visiting my son in hospital and his renal failure and then about my cancer operation tomorrow. He seemed a little taken aback and I thought, "I bet he wishes he had never asked!"

The Operation

The next day was the big one. I had been asked to arrive at the admissions ward for 7am and on arriving, joined a small queue of patients. After an hour or so, my name was called out and I was taken into a pre-theatre area. Surely the operation would

go ahead now; this was my hope. Kathy was with me and we sat talking and making jokes as we often do for about 20 minutes. We tend to have quite a black humour, probably influenced in Kathy's case by her life working as a nurse. It also helps defuse serious situations and I find makes the waiting less fearful. Finally, theatre technicians arrived and took me into the area where you meet the anaesthetist. He also reiterated all the things that might happen to me such as embolisms, cardiac events, etc! I once again felt so reassured! I then received an injection; I must admit I enjoyed the sensation of drifting off within seconds of the needle going into the vein ...

The next thing I remember was waking on the ward, probably about four hours later, and Kathy telling me that my surgeon had been up to see her and told her the operation had gone well. I had an uneventful night on the ward and although in some discomfort, the pain relief being administered was very effective. Later that morning, Kathy and her brother came in to see me and spent an hour or so entertaining me, although I still felt a bit woozy. Kathy came back again that evening and gave me an update on everything, including how many pheasants Cara had chased on her morning walk. We said our goodbyes and I settled down for the night, although as anyone who has been in hospital knows, you are woken every couple of hours to have your temperature and blood pressure etc. taken, so sleep is a rare commodity.

The second night in my hospital bed was not so good. There was a lot of activity on the ward and the nursing staff were seemingly rushed off their feet with either late admissions or patients developing problems through the evening period.
A man was admitted into the next bed to mine and he had developed pneumonia in addition to his abdominal condition. They connected him to a machine to aid his breathing. I felt for this chap and what he was going through, but the additional noise of the machine made sleeping only a remote possibility for me. Then, at about midnight, just as I was drifting into another world, the man in the bed opposite mine started vomiting. The problem was exacerbated because he had a gastric tube in place following a complicated bowel condition which had apparently been ongoing for several months. Vomiting is not pleasant at the best of times, but to witness this poor man trying to do so, whilst having a tube down his throat at the same time, was really distressing. I now felt as though my procedure was a piece of cake compared to what he was going through and the suffering he must have endured over not days or weeks but months. The culmination of noise and activity on the

ward in the early hours, being on morphine, this poor chap opposite and probably a delayed reaction to my own diagnosis and procedure, caused me to feel as though I was having a panic attack. I felt as though I was trapped on the ward and needed to escape. I managed to get out of bed and walk with all my tubes and drug infusion bags, which were attached to a drip stand, down the ward. A staff nurse stopped me and asked if she could help and I said I felt as though I was having a panic attack and needed to leave the ward. I thought to myself, "She probably thinks I am a bit mad, but I need to get out." I just wanted some peace and quiet. She said I could sit in the corridor outside the ward for 20 minutes or so, but not to go further afield! Well, the fresh countryside air wasn't going to happen, but this would be an improvement on the chaos going on in the ward. I was so pleased that she understood my need for some time out. It was such a sense of relief and I stayed for probably half an hour, just sitting in that relatively quiet corridor, thinking a myriad of thoughts.

I thought about how suddenly your life can change. One moment we are in a fairly predictable pattern of events and suddenly we have to face the harsh reality, that like a car breaking down, our bodies go wrong. However, as a rule people only start to contemplate this when it happens. I also reflected on our time in the Cotswolds and suddenly saw parallels between the snow and its silent arrival and my tumour that had begun silently, no warnings, both had grown in depth. In the case of the snow very quickly, with the cancer over a long period of time. It is only because we can't see a tumour growing in our colon that we are not aware of its presence. Until that it has reached the size where it can cause an obstruction or other symptoms*.

If we were unable to see the snow outside, we would only be aware of its presence if it reached such a depth that it made a thud as great chunks fell from the roof and hit the ground.

That was the equivalent of my colon obstructing. These are thoughts I had as I sat in that hospital corridor. It probably sounds weird, maybe it was because both events, the tumour and the snow made their presence felt at the same time.

When you go for your surgery, your focus is on the operation, the plumbing bit. The brain however has other ideas and reminds us that we are human beings with feelings and emotions; it tries to make sense of what we experience. I returned to the scenes of carnage on the ward, feeling a little calmer and more able to cope with my surroundings, and finally fell asleep.

In the morning, I spoke with the man in the bed opposite and asked how he was feeling after his traumatic night. He seemed very matter of fact about it and said he had had reactions before to his drip feed and after three months was accustomed to such events. I was only likely to remain in hospital for three to four days; three months would seem like a lifetime. This is the thing: whatever you experience in life, you will always meet someone who has had a worse time, suffered more and may continue to suffer. So, I never thought, "Why me?"; more likely, "Why not?"

The next day, I had some of my lines and tubes removed, the wound was less painful, and I had started to eat solids. I slept reasonably well on this Sunday evening and looked forward to Kathy's visit tomorrow afternoon and the prospect of going home. The ward also seemed less frantic and there was more of a sense of calmness. On Monday morning, I saw the surgical registrar who said, all being well, I could go home later that afternoon. Kathy came in to collect me, although we had to wait first for my drugs to arrive from the pharmacy. I had to have my final blood pressure, pulse and temperature taken before they would discharge me. Unfortunately, my oxygen saturation was low, my pulse was a little high (the law of Sod). I therefore then had to have an ECG (electrocardiogram) and wait for a doctor to interpret it. I can remember saying to Kathy that I was going home anyway! The nurse in her said to wait for the tests but in my own mind I was out of there whatever! The nurse then came back to redo my saturation levels. In the interim, I had been hyperventilating on purpose to get my oxygen levels back up; something I used to do when competitively swimming in my teenage years. I am not recommending anyone does this, but it did seem to have the desired effect, as when she remeasured my sats, they had gone up to about 97. A doctor approved my ECG and it was time to leave. I said my goodbyes and felt pleased to be going home to some peace and quiet.

Leaving the hospital and walking to the car, even though it was parked near the front entrance, was an uncomfortable experience. Previously I had only walked down the ward and to the toilet, so I soon realised that the operation wound site would take a little while to heal. Interestingly, they called the procedure "keyhole". All I can say is, it seemed a bloody big hole for a key, but in fairness the alternative is a full abdominal incision closed with staples, so I was grateful for the surgery I had!

We made the 15-minute drive home with me wincing at every bump in the road. However, was I pleased to get back to our cottage and sleep in a bed, where the only noises at night are of hooting owls. One interesting observation when I arrived home, was that Cara kept sniffing around my belly area where the operation had been, almost as though she knew something had gone on while I was in hospital; her nose was deciding exactly what.

My discomfort from the scar was reducing gradually and, under the advice given by my surgeon, I was to avoid putting any strain on the wound. No housework for me - what a result! Driving was also on hold for about a month or so; the criteria for resuming use of the car is apparently to be able to perform an emergency stop.

One procedure I did have to endure was a daily stabbing in the stomach area with a subcutaneous syringe to administer 'Clexane'. This drug, whose generic name is enoxaparin sodium, is used to prevent a post-operative deep-vein thrombosis or pulmonary embolism developing following certain types of surgery. I say a daily stabbing as the choice is either you commit hara-kiri, in other words, as in the Japanese self-styled disembowelment (do it yourself), or you get someone else to do it. With Kathy being a nurse, there is no way she was going to pass up on the opportunity to conduct this daily ritual; the prospect of stabbing me once a day brought a grin to her face. She almost seemed to revel at the prospect. She even asked me to score her on a 0-10 rating each time where 0 was pain free and 10 was agony. Fortunately, most scored between 2 and 4. Certainly, varying the target area helped, as repeated puncture wounds in the same area made it feel more tender. I endured the daily ritual for a month and, to be fair, the anticipation of each stabbing was worse than the actual event.

As time passed, I felt that my wound was repairing, feeling less uncomfortable and physically I started to feel well. The surgery really had made me feel so much better. What surprised me most was that, within a week, my poo was so normal. I expected with half of my large bowel missing that things would change. I hoped not to have diarrhoea, but did think my stools would be much looser, but it was as though I hadn't lost any bowel. I know one of the main functions of the large colon is the reabsorption of water, as well as calcium and elements like vitamin B12. So how does that work? What happens to that water? Does the small bowel make up for the loss of its big brother? It may be that most of the absorption of water is in the last couple of feet of the colon. I could ask Kathy, but I think she is getting bored of bowels (home and at work!)

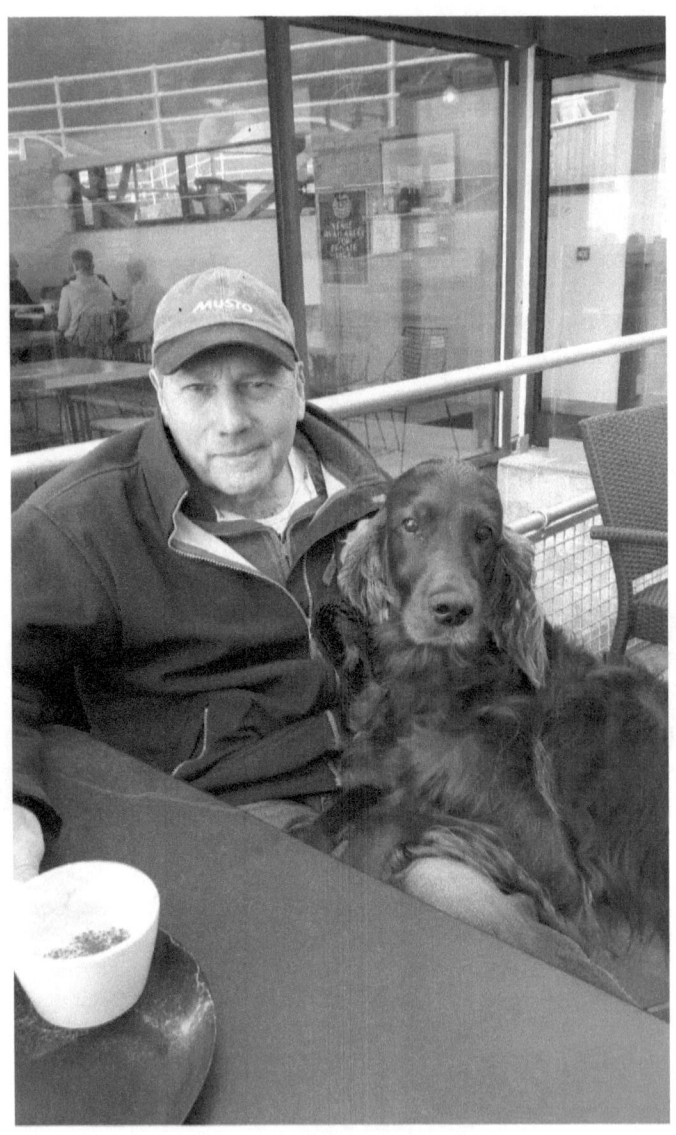

Cara and I having a coffee break

Post-Op follow-up

It was now time for my post-operative appointment with the surgeon. I was not sure what to expect. He would no doubt have information about the pathology of what he had removed including the lymph nodes. I felt a little apprehensive as I walked into his clinic room in the outpatients department, knowing that your prognosis and life expectancy is very dependent on the staging of your tumour and potential spread. Once again, it was so good to have Kathy by my side. I think even if you are living alone, it is so helpful to take a close friend or other relative to attend these appointments with you. You cannot always remember everything that is said in these consultations. Sometimes you fixate on one thing and forget to listen to everything else that is said, so having an extra pair of ears is a real advantage as well as feeling supported. Once he had asked how I had been since the surgery, he started to give me some feedback. He said he thought he had got everything out, meaning the cancer, and went on to say that because of the extent and location of the advanced tumour that had grown through the wall of my colon, there was only 0.7mm healthy margin on the surgery. The description of my tumour was, wait for it: "A moderately differentiated adenocarcinoma staged pT4a pN1b (3/14) EMVI +ve with an R1 resection - 0.7mm posterior resection margin". To say that's a bit of a mouthful is an understatement! It can seem bewildering and it's a lot to take in; all the nomenclature can seem very daunting and confusing. So, I will try to break that description down into chunks. The tumour, a pT4a, started its development in the mucosal lining of the colon, grown into the muscularis propria, a deeper, thick layer of muscle lining the colon. This normally contracts to force the contents of the intestines on its journey. The tumour had then grown through this muscular layer into tissues surrounding the colon and had reached the surface of the visceral peritoneum, which means it had grown through all the layers of the colon silently and without my knowledge. The pN1b (3/14) means that, of the 14 lymph nodes removed during surgery at the same time as the tumour, three were cancer positive. As for the EMVI +ve it stands for extramural vascular invasion and is a prognostic indicator in pT4 colorectal cancer. In other words, it is an indicator of survival and, put simply, your chances of survival are reduced by having it and as you can see, I had it.

The only good news seemed to be that the three cancer-positive nodes were close to the diseased part of the colon and the more distal nodes were not cancerous. However, the not so good news was that 0.7mm healthy margin meant there was very little room for error. I thought about 0.7mm; it didn't sound like much more than the width of a scalpel blade. Healthy margin means that in removing the tumour you naturally want to take a safe amount of healthy tissue with it, to be sure of getting all of the tumour out. The surgeon then said that in view of the three positive nodes and small healthy margin, I would receive a period of chemotherapy and will be referred to the Oncology department for an appointment, where I would get more specific advice. He did say that he felt he had removed everything and that he would expect the surgery to be curative. At least, I thought, we have finished on a positive, but I must admit I had my doubts with the 0.7mm, which over the coming weeks and months I would ponder on, even looking occasionally at a tape measure, to remind myself how little it was. Afterwards the surgeon introduced me to one of the colorectal specialist nurses, who spent a short period discussing chemotherapy and left me with a great wad of booklets to wade through - more bedtime reading. He said I would receive an appointment with an oncologist soon. We then went home and as usual with these things you reflect on everything. Overall, I felt positive, just that lingering doubt about the very small margin and the EMVI +ve. I also waded my way through all the information I had been given.

It was at about this time that Kathy decided she wanted a challenge. Why should I have all the fun! Her challenge was to raise money for Bowel Cancer West by running the Plymouth half marathon. The charity is dedicated to promoting research in the diagnosis and treatment of bowel cancer, education and training of the public and health professionals who care for bowel cancer patients across the West Country. It meant over a 12-week period that she would train to be able to run the 13 miles, which as someone who has never run any distance before would not be easy.

The 'Bad Boys'

After a couple of weeks, I received an appointment to see the oncologist - this was the bit I was not looking forward to. I was now feeling really well, and I knew the next step was to start a course of treatment that was going to make me progressively feel worse. There is a certain irony that the whole basis of chemotherapy is to try to eliminate any cancer cells in the blood or tissues but, in so doing, it kills lots of healthy ones as well, as the drugs are not able to differentiate. The body sustains this attack only because the healthy cells are able to reproduce faster than the cancer cells. I had obviously been reading about the various chemotherapy treatments in a package of booklets given to me by the specialist nurse who spoke to me after my last hospital appointment. The oncologist said he proposed a course of eight three-weekly cycles. I am thinking that's nearly six months! I asked how unpleasant the drugs would be and he said not as bad as some that we use. Another "Oh wonderful, how lucky am I!" moment popped into my head. What he was really saying was, be thankful some people have even worse treatments! The three-weekly cycles would consist of an intravenous drug infusion of oxaliplatin given on the oncology ward over two to three hours, followed by two weeks of oral capecitabine taken at home, and then a week drug-free to allow the body some recuperation from the onslaught. I was informed that I would have to have my bloods taken before each cycle.

The capecitabine, or 5-fluorouracil to give it its generic name, has its origins in chemical warfare and is related to mustard gas. Dr Stewart Francis Alexander, a lieutenant colonel who was an expert in chemical warfare, investigated the aftermath following the exposure of more than 1000 people to the SS John Harvey's secret cargo of mustard gas bombs in the 1920s. The autopsies of the victims suggested that profound lymphoid and myeloid suppression had occurred after the exposure. Dr Alexander theorised that since mustard gas all but ceased the division of certain types of somatic cells, whose nature was to divide fast, it could be put to use in helping to suppress the division of certain types of cancerous cells. So, forgive my emotional comparisons to the first war. What it does show is that even out of something developed to do serious harm in a war situation, a force for good can emerge. I would now get my very own sustained mustard gas attack, albeit in tablet form for the next six months! I was informed that I would start treatment in a week's time. I could hardly wait!

I now knew what my chemo regime was and what nasty substances would be used to fight any remaining cancer cells. I googled as most of us do these days and read some of the personal accounts that were posted. I also read all the chemo literature on possible and probable side effects. I suppose I looked on this treatment a bit like we view the wearing of seat belts or installing of air bags in our cars. There may not be any cancer left in my body after the surgery, you may not have an accident in your car, or you might, and I might have cancer cells in my blood stream, in which case you need the protection. I knew of people who had decided they didn't want to take up the chemo option, because they didn't want to feel rubbish and that the chances of their cancer recurring would only be improved by roughly 10%. It becomes a bit like gambling - what are the odds of my survival without the chemo and what are they with? I decided having already established that I had about a 50% chance of surviving five years with the chemo, it seemed to be a no-brainer; how could I afford not to have it?

Well, the time had come. My first cycle of chemo was to take place, with the infusion at the hospital. I arrived at the chemotherapy ward with Kathy and was told to take a seat and wait to be called. Looking around at other patients, you are reminded that you are one of many people with a cancer or leukaemia diagnosis. All adult age groups represented here, men and women, some looking very ill, some women with head scarfs, presumably because of hair loss. Others you would not know to look at them that they had anything wrong with them. After half an hour, I was called through by one of the nurses, weighed and taken to a unit with about eight beds. The oncology nurse was a real character and really funny, which did help to put me at my ease. I was asked which hand I wanted to be cannulated and then was told to place the hand in a dish of warm water, presumably to cause the veins to stand out more. A cannula was put into my vein and attached to a bag of the drug oxaliplatin.

I was given an injection of steroid which I was informed would give you a funny feeling in your bum. It did and was a sort of warm tickly feeling. Don't ask me why it does this, but it does. Then the chemo drug was switched on and would deliver its contents over two to three hours. I was given a heated pillow to place my hand on and was told this would make the process less uncomfortable. I realised after about half an hour what they meant, as the hand that was being infused started to sting, rather like what you would experience with nettles. As the time progressed this stinging became more apparent. It wasn't agony; it was just very uncomfortable. I thought this agent is stinging because it's attacking the cells around the vein into which it was being delivered. I contented myself by thinking if it finds any cancer cells, I hope it gives them hell. My understanding of how these chemo agents work is that they prevent cancer cells reproducing at the point where they normally divide. Often more than one chemo agent may be used as they will act at different stages of the reproduction cycle or they may induce cell death, called apoptosis, literally causing cancer cells to commit suicide. Whenever I was having a chemo infusion or taking chemo tablets, I tried to visualise this process Imagining the chemical agents as fighters with swords slashing these unwelcome cancer visitors, or cancer cells leaping to their death off the Tamar bridge, rather than face destruction by the chemical attack. You can see I do have a rather vivid imagination. Once the chemo agent had run through, an alarm would go off and the nurse returned to attach a flushing agent, the whole process taking about three hours. Well, that was my first cycle started and apart from the stinging during the infusion it wasn't too bad. My wrist did continue to feel sore for quite a while after the procedure. On leaving the hospital, bearing in mind it was February, Kathy reminded me to cover my mouth with a scarf and to wear some woollen gloves that I had brought with me. I had been informed that on breathing in the cold air following the infusion it could cause you to choke! Another lovely side-effect! The scarf helped prevent the cold air causing this effect. It is documented in all the information you receive. The effect normally wears off after a few hours; keeping the cold air out really does prevent the reaction. The gloves are advised to be worn to reduce any peripheral neuropathy in the hands, a drug side effect. Once home we sat down to eat. As it was getting late, we had just decided on a jacket potato with cheese, a favourite snack of mine. I bit into it and exclaimed loudly, "Arrghh, that's awful!" I hadn't realised the chemo would affect my taste buds so quickly. It tasted like soap mixed with papier mache. I was soon to realise that cold drinks or chilled food from the refrigerator was not an option. You experience the same sort of choking feeling as breathing in cold air after your chemo infusion. Even tap water was too cold to swallow and had to be warmed up before I could drink it. I soon realised that I could only really taste and enjoy strongly flavoured things. I have never eaten so many chillies and curries as during that six months!

We left the hospital having been given a supply of the oral chemo agent (the chemo nurse had called these tablets, "Bad boys!" even writing it on the box). In addition, I was given drugs to treat any side effects such as vomiting or diarrhoea, a supply of steroids to be taken for the first three days of each cycle and a cream to rub into your feet as hand-foot syndrome is often a side effect of the oral capecitabine. Neuropathy of the hands is a common side effect which can be permanent, affecting you long after you finish your chemo. If you touch anything metallic it feels like your hands are holding a block of ice and your instinct is to drop the item, very weird. I often wore gloves to hold a knife and fork after my infusion for this same reason. You do get the odd stare especially if you are having a meal out in public. Another side effect of these agents is that they impact your immune system making it easier for you to pick up infections or colds. You are advised to avoid being near children and pregnant women when on chemo and to flush the toilet twice after use to avoid any risk to other users. I calculated that by the end of the eighth cycle, I would have swallowed nearly 900 'bad boys'!

At the risk of boring you with details of each cycle, what I will say is that every cycle is preceded by blood tests and an appointment with the oncologist to check you are on the right dose of infusion and to gauge how you are standing up to the side effects. I do remember seeing the oncologist prior to my starting the third cycle and saying that I was finding it easier than I had expected. He replied, "Wait till you get to your fifth cycle. It does get worse because the effects are cumulative!" I was later to discover that he was right about that.

I never had any sickness or diarrhoea, but I did feel nauseous quite often. I did have a metallic taste in my mouth and most food was not enjoyable, often tasteless. I noticed my poo was not the usual colour but a hideous grey, also caused by the chemo agents. My hands were affected by the neuropathy, but the most impactful side effect is the fatigue. It progressively got worse with each cycle, making you feel worn out all the time, even when you haven't done anything. I will try to describe the difference between tiredness and fatigue: with tiredness you can have a nap or sleep and wake up feeling refreshed. With fatigue you take a nap or sleep and wake up still feeling worn out.

Sunshine in France

It was after my 4th cycle that Kathy ran her half marathon in Plymouth. I went to the event to give my support and it was a beautiful day, although perhaps a little too warm for running. The charity she was raising funds for, 'Bowel Cancer West', had a stand at the event and I met the chairman and founder, who is also the surgeon that performed my operation. Once again, I thanked him for all he had done for me, commending him on his surgical skills. Kathy completed the run in a respectable time and in the process raised nearly £900 for the charity. She was delighted and once again I had good reason to be proud of her.

We had planned to take a short holiday to France before I reached the stage of being continually fatigued. We felt we needed to escape the monotony of everything revolving around the cycles of chemo and needed a change of scenery. We coincided our trip with my drug-free respite week which always followed the two weeks of chemo and was generally when I would feel better. We had arranged to spend two nights in a lovely cave suite, a unique suite of rooms hewn long ago into the rock beside a bell-topped presbytery. It was situated in a small village called Rochecorbon in the Loire valley, not far from Tours. The following two nights we were to spend in the village of Sarthe, just south of Le Mans. That was the plan, but unfortunately the best laid plans of mice and men and all that ... We had booked to travel by ferry from Poole to Cherbourg. We left our home the day before so that we could stay in the small inn that I had stayed at previously when visiting my son in hospital. It would break the journey and make sure we were in Poole for the 8am sailing. We had a really nice night at The Greyhound, the room was delightful, and the food and ales were very good. We left the inn at about 6.30am, which meant we had to forgo a cooked breakfast. Kindly, the staff had left a buffet breakfast which was more than adequate to keep us going for a few hours. However, on arriving at the ferry port in Poole, we were informed that due to a lightning strike by the French operators, all crossings from Poole had been cancelled for the day. We couldn't believe it. At first, they said, "We can get you on a crossing from Plymouth"! We had spent the previous day driving from our home near Plymouth, so the prospect of driving all the way back seemed like a nightmare. Finally, they agreed we could cross from Portsmouth, only an hour's drive from Poole. The problem was, the later sailing meant arriving late in Cherbourg and so we had to cancel our first night in the cave suite, as our

44

arrival time would have been ridiculously late. We apologised to the would-be hosts and explained that we had no control over the actions of the French ferry operators. They were very understanding. We got off the ferry at 22.30 and drove for an hour looking for somewhere to stay without success; it wasn't helped by us losing our way and our Google Maps not working on our phones. We thought with hindsight we should have just pitched up at a hotel in Cherbourg. Eventually we arrived in a village near to Bayeux, famous for its tapestries, everywhere seemed closed. Kathy at this point was losing the will to live and when we arrived at a small car park, she was close to tears, thinking we were going to have to spend the night in our mini. Suddenly I saw a light in a window and the outline of a woman drawing the curtains closed. Kathy and I leapt from the car and rushed to the door of what we could now confirm as a small private hotel. The lady answered and we asked if she had a chamber. She said she had and with relief we said to each other, whatever it's like we will have it! The room was typically French provincial, modest but clean. The hotel owner was very friendly and with Kathy's basic grasp of French we managed to understand each other. We slept really well and had a great continental breakfast the next morning.

We left after breakfast and drove south. About an hour south of Le Mans we hit a storm with torrential rain and for a while had to drive at 20 miles an hour until it had passed, finally reaching Tours at about 16.30. Here we got lost and ended up having to make our way to the tourist office to get advice on how to find the tiny village of Rochecorbon. We probably spent an hour in Tours, but with new advice on the best route, found our way to our destination by about 18.00. It was worth all the trouble - a really pretty little village and when we arrived at our hosts' property, we were very impressed. It was like a small chateau in a walled enclosure, very historic but beautifully kept and they were such a charming and friendly couple. They showed us our cave suite and we were flabbergasted; it was simply beautiful, the like of which we shall probably never see again. The way the rooms had been built into this white rock which just gleamed was something to behold. The décor was so tasteful and everything you would need for your stay was to be found. They invited us for an evening pre-dinner drink in their chateau and we chatted about all and sundry as they spoke excellent English. They recommended a restaurant which we could walk to and we thanked them for their hospitality and said we would see them for breakfast.

Once again, we got lost trying to find this restaurant, even though it was only a 15-minute walk away. Getting lost seemed to be a feature of this holiday but eventually, after several detours, we arrived. We had an excellent meal and chose a fine wine to accompany the meal from their ground-floor cellar, which we were encouraged to explore.

The next morning, we had a lovely breakfast in our hosts' home before saying our goodbyes and adding that we would return one day and spend two- or three-nights next time. We had two more enjoyable days in Sarthe, visiting Le Lude Chateau, Le Mans car museum and the old city area of Le Mans, known as the Plantagenet city because of its twelfth-century origins, which is simply amazing. I have had many holidays driving through France in the past and well remember one trip in 1969 when I had driven back from

Toulouse to London in a mini with no front disk brakes. They had worn down to the metal and I had to rely on the use of gears and my handbrake operating on the back brakes to slow down. I just didn't have the money to get them replaced at a French garage! however, I survived. Now it was back to reality, and the day after getting home it was back to the hospital to start Cycle Five.

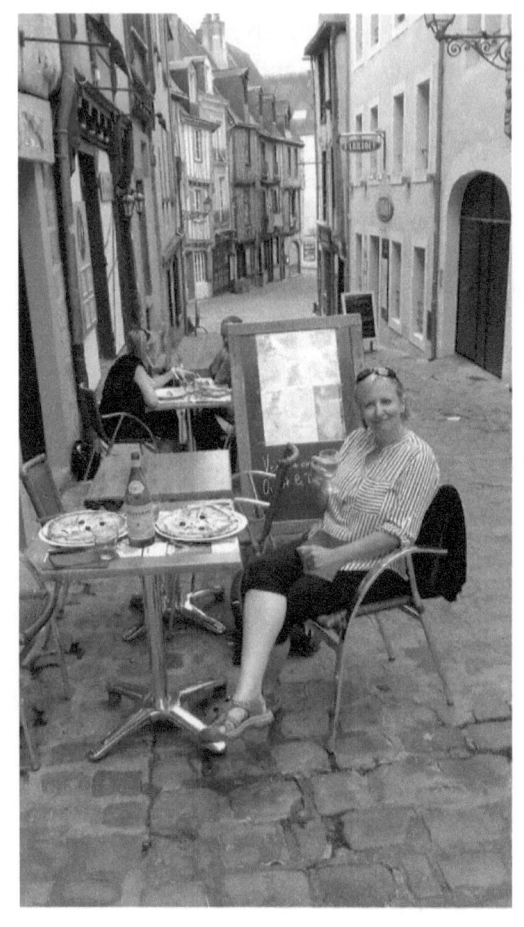

Lunch in Le -mans old city

Say Goodbye to the 'Bad Boys'

The break in France had been a good decision; however, as I got into this cycle, I realised the oncologist's words about the cumulative effect of the chemo were coming true. I felt totally wiped out and would get breathless just from walking up a nearby hill in our village with Cara. She seemed to understand something was not quite right and slowed her pace to match mine. I had also by now accepted that food was only going to have any taste if it was spiced up, so curry was good and adding chilli flakes to various other meals at least made them more enjoyable. As my hand neuropathy progressively got worse, the oncologist reduced the dose of my infusion for my fifth cycle by 20%, as they were concerned about permanent damage. During this cycle, my week's break from chemo did not give me any apparent respite from the fatigue, which just seemed endless.

One bizarre, if not interesting observation I had on chemo treatment; followed a short walk with Cara on Dartmoor. It was during a warm spell in June and after returning home I noticed a small blood scab on my ankle. I assumed that I had caught it on a bramble and didn't think any more about it. However, a couple of days later, Kathy noticed it and had a closer look. She said, 'that's not a blood scab it's a tick'. She carefully removed it and when we examined it, realised it was shrivelled up, strangely malformed and quite dead. Normally if we ever found any ticks on Cara; especially if they had been undetected for a few days, they would be bloated with blood, round and a shiny silvery-black colour. We concluded that in drawing my blood, the tick had literally bitten off more than it could chew. The tick had also taken on the toxic chemo agents circulating in my blood stream and they had obliterated the offending parasite. I find ticks quite disgusting creatures and could not disguise my pleasure in the fate that had befallen this unwelcome visitor. On relating this story to the Oncology registrar at my next appointment she seemed rather amused by the episode, if not a little in awe of her potent chemical armoury!

During June, Kathy received some amazing news: she was to receive a prestigious nursing award, called the Dr Kate Granger Award, for compassionate care. This is recognised both nationally and internationally and she was to be the sole recipient in her hospital trust. We then discovered that one of her consultant gastroenterologists had nominated her for the award and had been supported by many of her patients. It was so good to share in her excitement and to be able to attend the presentation at the postgraduate centre of the hospital with her mum. The award was made by the CEO of the hospital and Dr Granger's husband. His wife had contracted a rare form of cancer whilst in her late 20s. She set the award up because she realised that during her treatment she was often treated without compassion, those administering care often not even introducing themselves when they took blood or administered drugs. Unfortunately, Dr Granger died a couple of years later and her husband has continued her work gaining notoriety and making a difference in attitude towards compassionate care. One particularly funny moment was when the photographer at the award ceremony said to Kathy, "How brilliant that both your mum and dad could attend the event." I should point out her mum was there, but her dad wasn't; he was referring to me! Kathy is some 20 years my junior and a very youthful looking 50-year-old. She did put him right and I saw him redden up and could just feel his embarrassment. This award ceremony had been a welcome distraction, and I was over the moon for my hero.

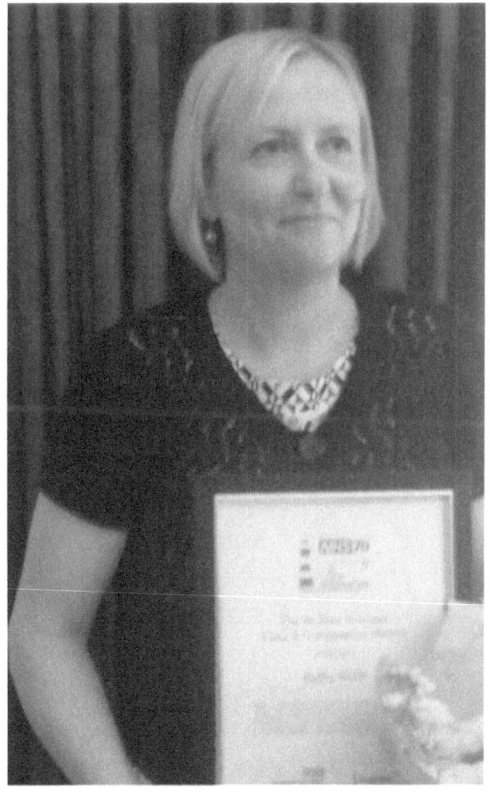

Kathy at her award ceremony

It was now time to start my sixth cycle of chemo. After the infusion, the oncologist said that would be my last infusion of oxaliplatin. Despite the reduced dose, he still had concerns about my hands and the risk of permanent damage. He said the majority of patients did not go beyond six cycles because of side effects. I must admit, since cycle five the signs of neuropathy in my hands were continuing into the third week of each cycle when I was drug free, whereas in previous cycles it had worn off during the third week. He continued saying that most of the benefit from the drug in combating any potential cancer cells would have been achieved now and I would not be significantly disadvantaged in not having the last two cycles. I was however to continue with the oral chemo. I went home feeling glad that I would not have to go further with the infusions; my hands had taken a battering and would now be left in peace. However, I had also reached a point where I was fed up with taking the oral medication. The combined effects of fatigue, nausea and metallic taste made just swallowing eight of these 'bad boys' a daily effort. I waited till I was alone and threw the remaining tablets in the pedal bin. They were still in their metal foil and I made sure Kathy wouldn't see them, placing them under other rubbish. I thought if six cycles were enough for the infusion, it would have to be enough for the tablets. I had reached the end of the line and was fed up feeling so awful all the time. I just wanted to get back to feeling well again.

It didn't take Sherlock Holmes long to find out what I had done! That evening Kathy was emptying the pedal bin and saw the shiny metal foils containing 112 tablets, my two-week supply.

Once she had removed the previous night's lasagne leftovers and other debris from the metal foils, she reinstated the medicine in our cupboard. She then used her clinical and most persuasive manner to convince me of the folly in not seeing out cycles seven and eight: "You're taking them, no arguments!" Another six weeks and it would all be finished. I could get my life back on track and I would have given this derivative of 'mustard gas' its best chance of nuking the enemy. Maybe a part of me wanted her to find those tablets in the bin because I needed Kathy to convince me to continue. I did continue and I finished cycles seven and eight … bloody hooray! On Friday 27th July I took my last eight tablets and breathed an almighty sigh of relief. I was told not to expect to feel fully back to normal for about six months, but that I would see a gradual improvement over the coming weeks. Apparently, it takes that long for your immune system to recover and for your white cells to start reproducing at their normal rate. The next day Kathy suggested we have a celebratory meal at our local pub, not an offer I was going to refuse. What was so nice was that the manager, whom we knew well, had reserved a table for us and had covered it in silver stars and messages of support as well as party poppers, balloons and a bottle of prosecco. We had one of the best nights ever, a delicious curry that I could taste and a lot of laughs.

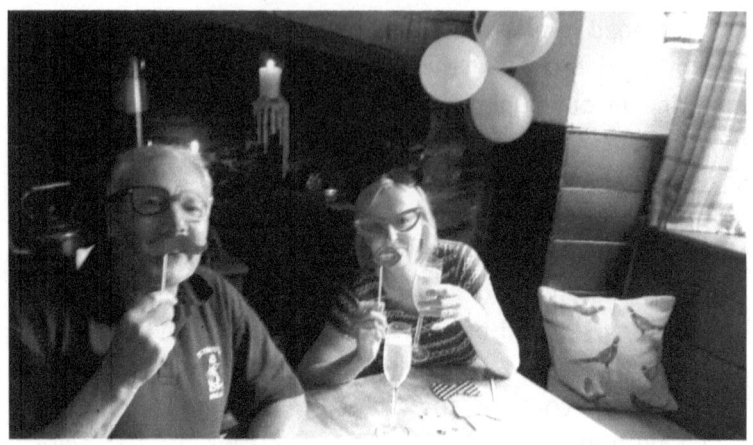

Celebrating the end of chemo

Now that I had finished taking all the chemo agents, as the weeks ticked by, I started feeling less fatigued. The metallic taste disappeared and my ability to enjoy the real taste of food had returned. The only lingering side effect was the neuropathy in my hands and also now in my feet. In fact, my feet felt odd, as though I was walking barefooted with wet sponges attached. On one occasion I fell down the stairs, as my feet just were not giving me the normal sure footing and feedback that you take for granted. Luckily, I didn't do any damage to myself but did break a small oak table in the process which I had fallen onto. Kathy did look over the banister at the almighty crash and said, "Oh God, you haven't broken the table, have you?" Never mind any damage I might have sustained! It taught me a lesson and am more aware now of this limitation.

Four months after finishing chemo, I restarted my part-time job with the out-of-hours GP service and was now feeling the best I had for a long time. However, on reaching my 72nd Birthday, some 8 months later I did finally retire from this part-time job. It was time to just relax and take life easy. I had enjoyed my three years in the job. In addition to all the seriousness of dealing with some real tragedy and sadness amongst the more mundane medical issues, there had also been some very funny moments.

I well remember the GP, who just happened to be my own GP, who finding he needed to use a patient's toilet, locked the door and was then unable to unlock it. He called to me out of the toilet window, as I waited in the emergency vehicle outside and I had to break the door down to get him out. The 83-year-old patient had agreed to my physical intervention. The prospect of me wrecking her previously immaculately painted toilet door, was no reason to restrain my shoulder charge!

A visit to confirm an expected death at a Nursing home, became the case of the mysterious disappearing body. When we arrived, no one could find the deceased patient, who had passed away some 5 or 6 hours previously. There had been a change of shift and it seems the information was not passed on. The doctor eventually found out that the body had already been taken to the undertakers, without confirmation of death and signing of a death certificate. As the undertakers was now well and truly closed, a visit had to be made the next day and the coroner informed. When the lady was fortunately confirmed to be dead and a certificate duly signed.

Then there was the lady who was disabled and deaf. Her carer had rung 111 to say she thought she was confused and not herself; she had a 'key safe' but our notes did not have the code! We tried phoning and knocking the door, without success, not surprising as she was deaf! It becomes a welfare issue when a patient is thought to be at home but cannot be raised, they may have collapsed etc. It is then incumbent on the doctor in these situations to gain entry. Our only choice was to call the fire brigade to access the property. They arrived at midnight, blue lighting in a full-size fire engine. They were all helmeted and after gaining entry through an open bedroom window, discovered the lady awake in bed. You can just imagine her bewilderment, feeling unwell but minding her own business, when a six-foot helmeted fireman suddenly appeared at her bedroom window! Apparently, she was delighted with all the attention. This was followed by teas all round courtesy of one of the firemen. The GP confirmed the lady was in good spirits and only in need of some antibiotics for a urinary infection. We said all our goodbyes to the assembled congregation and headed off to the next victim!

This gentleman with a respiratory infection living on Dartmoor, had called back to 111 asking if we could pick up some fish and chips on route at 01.00 in the morning. To find a fish and chip shop open in the middle of a city after 22.00 is a challenge let alone in the middle of Dartmoor, we know that doctors can sometimes work miracles but even Jesus would struggle with this one. We had not been informed of this update so on arrival the GP had assessed the patient, deciding he needed an antibiotic and some steroids. He came back to the vehicle to ask me to dispense the drugs and reported that the patient seemed more concerned that he hadn't got his fish and chips!

There was the occasion when a young female GP went in to see a youngish patient who had a lethal combination of dogs and rabbits running around her house. When the GP came back to the vehicle she looked and walked in a very uneasy way. I got out and asked her if everything was ok. She said the house was covered in faeces and she had only realised after putting her bag down and stepping into some freshly laid deposits. We drove to a petrol station opposite the house, I bought a shed load of baby wipes and we spent the next 20 minutes cleaning up the doctor's shoes and her bag. I could go on and maybe there is a book to be written, but with GP's frequently falling asleep in the vehicle, it brings home how hard and what long hours they work. After 23.00 the service in the Plymouth area has one vehicle and one GP for home visits, to cover over 400 square miles. Resources are stretched and if this makes you think twice whether you need a visit or can make your own way to the 'out of hours' treatment centre, then I am glad I mentioned it.

The Transplant

I had visited my son several times over the period since going onto chemo, in particular when he had the surgery to remove his diseased kidneys. He had ended up having both of his kidneys removed in two separate operations over a three-month period and then went onto dialysis. These operations were not straightforward as each kidney had grown in size to over 5kg, the size of a large baby, and had become attached to other internal organs. He endured a really tough time, far worse than I had experienced. During September, he received a call to go to Portsmouth as a kidney had been found to be a near-perfect match. It was a cadaver kidney which was brought down from London. I cannot tell you how wonderful it was to hear this news. I received a text from him to say he was on his way to the hospital. We dared to hope the kidney would be a life saver and not be rejected. I am pleased to report his new kidney is working really well and he is better than he has been for many years. He started a new job five months after the transplant and the transformation in his health is quite amazing. This was such a relief for all of us, I can tell you, but my thoughts and thanks also went out to the person who had to die in order for my son to live. Such is the world of organ donation.

The Future

It is now eighteen months since my cancer surgery, and I feel great. I was recently given the all-clear following a colonoscopy, scans and biopsies. One procedure I had not previously had, was a PET scan (positron emission tomography). It produces three-dimensional images. It differs from a CT scan in that it can detect cancer at a molecular level. You are given an injection of a radioactive dye which contains a sugar-based compound. Cancer cells are more greedy than normal cells so they will compete more successfully to take up the radioactive sugar and be stained by the dye. This makes them more visible on the scan. It is odd when the nurse brings in a container with the radioactive symbol on it. They inject you with its contents whilst they are wearing radioactive protection. They then retreat for half an hour saying, "I have to go as I don't want to be irradiated". I suppose because of the frequency of their exposure you can understand why, but it is still unnerving. I will probably only feel totally out of the woods if my next scan in six months' time is found to be clear. I would then be off the radar for five years with no more hospital visits.

It has been a journey and one of many that people are making every day. I have a friend who had significant symptoms of bowel cancer for over a year, a colonoscopy was performed eventually but much later than should have been the case despite numerous GP visits. I didn't have any real symptoms until I started obstructing, so the symptomatic course of this disease may vary for individuals, particularly dependant on where the tumour is located in the bowel. I also recall just 2 months prior to my diagnosis being admitted to Hospital with pneumonia and sepsis, the man opposite me on the ward had been admitted for a severe chest infection, whilst having investigations he was diagnosed with lung cancer. He seemed to take it quite well, but I remember his family visiting and getting very upset at the news. I thought how terrible for him and his relatives, little realising I already had a growing tumour that in eight weeks my family and I would be dealing with.   C'est la vie.

Every two minutes someone in the UK is diagnosed with one of more than 100 different types of cancer. One in 14 men and one in 19 women will be diagnosed with bowel cancer in their lifetime. Some 42,000 people are diagnosed with this form of cancer every year. It is treatable and curable, especially if diagnosed early. I was lucky, despite having an advanced tumour that had spread to neighbouring lymph nodes. If Kathy had not been so on the ball, I dread to think of what would have happened. I feel positive about the future and in writing this I aim to give others going through this difficult process strength and determination to carry on.

I realise not everyone is as lucky as I am to have got this far. I am sure many sufferers will go through similar feelings and thoughts at times during their own journeys; sometimes knowing that others have been through it too can really help. One thing I feel compelled to say is having been through this experience I am reminded that life which we can all take for granted is fragile. It has heightened my enjoyment of whatever time I may have left. Savour the moment, enjoy your environment and feel more engaged with life.

I remember my very wise Tibetan Lama, Khenpo Lekshey once saying life is like a dream so make sure it's a pleasant one. Bad things happen, over which you have no control, but how you react to those things is down to us as individuals.

The snow and my cancer, both have disappeared, no trace for now, almost as though they had never existed. Whether that remains the case only time will provide the answer. If it snows again next winter on our annual pilgrimage to the Cotswolds, I will not be complaining, only too pleased to be there to witness it.

All profits from the sale of this book with be donated to

the

Bowel Cancer West Charity

Glossary

Anaemia: a condition in which there is a deficiency of red cells or of haemoglobin in the blood resulting in pallor and weariness.

Caecal Tumour: implies right sided colonic cancer in the caecum. The patient usually presents with unexplained pain in the right iliac fossa or general symptoms such as anaemia, malaise and weakness.

Cancer: a condition where cells in a specific part of the body grow and reproduce uncontrollably. The cancerous cells can invade and destroy surrounding healthy tissue including organs.

Cancer staging is the process of determining the extent to which a cancer has developed, by growing and spreading. Current practice is to assign a number from T1 – T4. The higher the number the more advanced.

Cannulation: intravenous (iv) cannulation is a technique in which a cannula is placed inside a vein to provide access. This allows for samples of blood to be taken as well as the administrations of fluids, medication, nutrition, chemotherapy and blood products.

Capecitabine: is a chemotherapy drug. It is used to treat many types of cancer including breast, colon, rectal, stomach, oesophageal and pancreatic cancers. It is used In tablet form.

Cardiac event: refers to any incidents that may cause damage to the heart muscle.

Chemotherapy: is a cancer treatment where medication is used to kill cancer cells. There are many different types of chemotherapy, but they all work in a similar way. They stop cancer cells reproducing, which prevents them from growing and spreading in the body.

Colonoscopy: is the endoscopic examination of the large bowel (colon) with a fibre optic camera.

CT scan: a computerised tomography (CT) scan uses x-rays and a computer to create detailed images of the inside of the body.

EMVI extra mural vascular invasion: used to evaluate the severity of vascular invasion in bowel cancer. **EMVI +ve**: indicates the presence of this prognostic indicator.

Inflammatory Bowel Disease: A term used to describe two conditions: ulcerative colitis (uc) and crohn's disease (cd); both of which are long term conditions that involve inflammation of the gut. They differ in that uc only affects the colon (large intestine) whereas cd can affect any part of the digestive tract from mouth to anus.

Ferritin: s a blood cell protein that contains iron. A ferritin test helps to understand how much iron your body is storing.

FIT test: is a screening test for colon cancer. It tests for hidden blood in the stool, which can be an early sign of cancer. FIT only detects human blood from the lower intestines.

ECG: electrocardiogram, a simple test that is used to check your hearts rhythm and electrical activity.

Gastroenterology: the study of the gastrointestinal tract.

Gastroscopy: a procedure where a thin flexible tube is used to look into the gullet, stomach and first part of the intestine.

gFOBT: a test that checks for hidden blood in the stool. This test is being replaced by the FIT test.

Hand – foot syndrome: side effect of chemotherapy causing redness swelling and pain in the hands and feet.

Keyhole surgery or laparoscopy is a type of surgical procedure that allows the surgeon to access inside of the abdomen, without having to make large incisions.

Oesophagus: the gullet.

Oxygen saturation: levels of oxygen in the blood stream.

Oxaliplatin: a chemotherapy drug used for the treatment of bowel cancer.

PET scan: positron emission tomography. Imaging that allows your doctor to check for diseases in your body even at a molecular level.

Peripheral neuropathy: damage to the nerves in the body's extremities, particularly the hands and feet.

Polycystic kidney disease: genetic disorder where the kidney grows multiple cysts.

Pulmonary embolism: a blockage in one of the pulmonary (lung) arteries, caused by a blood clot.